MW00513282

Anti-inflammatory diet Cookbook for women after 50

Smart Recipes for Busy people who want to eat well, lose weight fast, heal immune system and Restore Health

Polly Arnold

© Copyright 2021 - All rights reserved

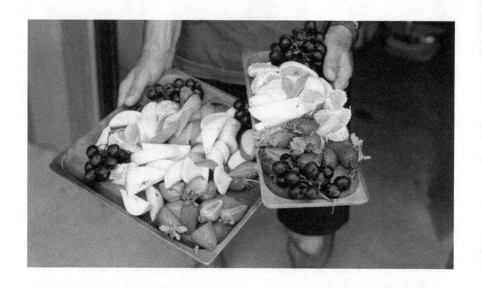

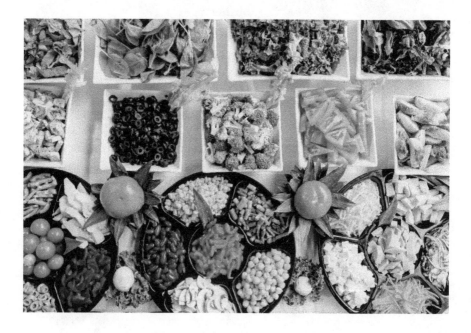

Table Of Contents

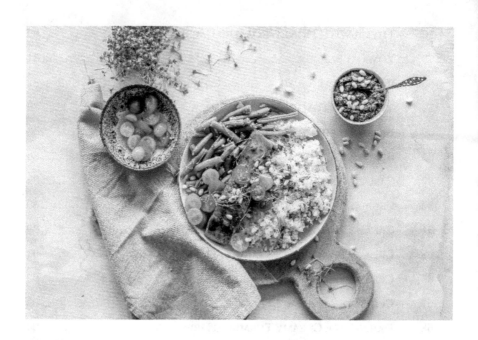

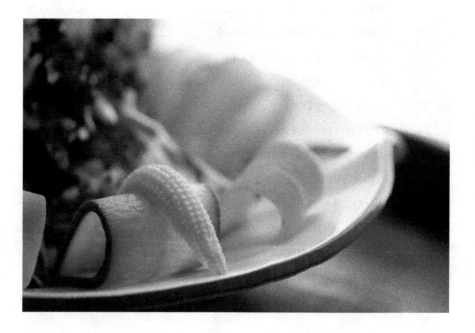

<u>Recipes</u>

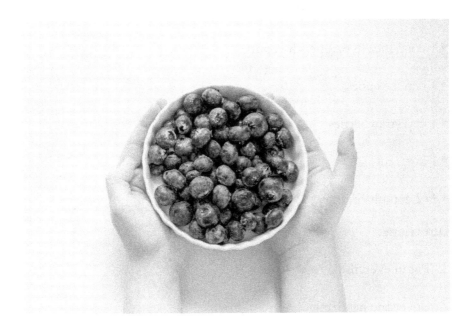

1. TRIPLE FRUIT SMOOTHIE

Time To Prepare: ten minutes

Time to Cook: 0 minutes **Yield:** Servings 1

Ingredients:

- 1 banana, peeled and chopped

- 1 container (8 oz.) peach yogurt

- 1 cup ice cubes

- 1 cup strawberries

- 1 kiwi, cut

- 1/2 cup blueberries • 1/2 cup orange juice

Directions:

1. Put in everything to a blender jug.

2. Cover the jug firmly.

3. Blend until the desired smoothness is achieved. Serve and enjoy!

Nutritional Info: Calories: 124 , Fat: 0.4 g , Protein: 5.6 g , Carbohydrates: 8 g , Fiber: 2.3 g

2. TROPICAL MANGO COCONUT SMOOTHIE

Time To Prepare: five minutes

Time to Cook: 0 minutes **Yield:** Servings 2

Ingredients:

- ½ cup of canned coconut milk

- ½ cup of fresh orange juice

- 1 ½ cups of frozen mango

- 1 ½ tsp of honey

- 1 medium frozen banana • 1 tbsp. of fresh lemon juice

Directions:

1. Mix the smoothie ingredients in your high-speed blender.

2. Pulse the ingredients a few times to cut them up.

3. Combine the mixture on the highest speed setting for thirty to 60 seconds.

4. Pour into glasses and serve.

Nutritional Info: Calories: 354 kcal , Protein: 6.7 g , Fat: 18.09 g , Carbohydrates: 47.42 g

3. TROPICAL PINEAPPLE KIWI SMOOTHIE

Time To Prepare: five minutes

Time to Cook: 0 minutes **Yield:** Servings 2 **Ingredients:**

- 1 ½ cup of frozen pineapple

- 1 cup of canned full-fat coconut milk

- 1 ripe kiwi; peeled and chopped

- 1 tsp of spirulina powder

- 3 tsp of lime juice

- 6 to 8 ice cubes

Directions:

1. Mix the smoothie ingredients in your high-speed blender.

2. Pulse the ingredients a few times to cut them up.

3. Combine the mixture on the highest speed setting.

4. Pour into glasses and serve.

Nutritional Info: Calories: 480 kcal , Protein: 7.38 g , Fat: 31.92 g , Carbohydrates: 48.35 g

4. TURMERIC AND GINGER TONIC

Time To Prepare: five minutes

Time to Cook: ten minutes **Yield:** Servings 4

Ingredients:

• 1/8 teaspoon cayenne pepper

• 2 tablespoons grated, fresh ginger

• 2 tablespoons grated, fresh turmeric

• 6 cups water

• Juice of 2 lemons

• Maple syrup or honey to taste

• The rind of 2 lemons, peeled

Directions:

1.   Put in water, ginger, turmeric, cayenne pepper, and lemon rind into a deep cooking pan.

2.   Put the deep cooking pan on moderate to high heat. (Do not boil) 3. Once the mixture is hot, remove from heat.

4. Strain into 4 mugs. Put in honey and lemon juice and stir.

5. Serve warm.

Nutritional Info: Calories: 48 kcal , Protein: 2.28 g , Fat: 1.81 g , Carbohydrates: 7.03 g

5. TURMERIC DELIGHT

Time To Prepare: five minutes

Time to Cook: 0 minutes **Yield:** Servings 2

Ingredients:

• ¼ Teaspoon Ginger

• ½ Teaspoon Cinnamon

• 1 Banana, Sliced

• 1 Tablespoon Lemon Juice, Fresh - 1 Teaspoon Turmeric

• 2 Cups Yogurt, Plain & Whole Milk

• 2 Teaspoons Honey, Raw

Directions:

Combine all ingredients into a blender then blend until the desired smoothness is achieved. **Nutritional Info:** Calories: 234 , Protein: 9.3 Grams , Fat: 8.2 Grams , Carbohydrates: 33.5 Grams

6. TURMERIC HOT CHOCOLATE

Time To Prepare: five minutes

Time to Cook: ten minutes **Yield:** Servings 2

Ingredients:

- 1/8 tsp. cayenne pepper, optional

- 1/8 tsp. pepper

- 2 cups milk

- 2 tsp. ground turmeric

- 3 tbsp. cacao or cocoa powder

- 4 tsp. coconut oil

- 4 tsp. honey

Directions:

1. Put in milk, turmeric, cocoa, and coconut oil into a deep cooking pan. Put the deep cooking pan on moderate heat. Coconut oil and pepper are added because it helps to absorb the turmeric.

2. Whisk regularly until well blended.

3. When it starts to boil, remove from heat. Put in honey, cayenne pepper, and pepper and whisk well.

4. Split into 2 cups before you serve.

Nutritional Info: Calories: 339 kcal , Protein: 12.76 g , Fat: 21.19 g , Carbohydrates: 30.35 g

7. TURMERIC TEA

Time To Prepare: five minutes

Time to Cook: fifteen minutes **Yield:** Servings 2

Ingredients:

- ½ teaspoon ground ginger

- ½ teaspoon turmeric powder

- ½ tsp ground cinnamon

- 2 cups water

- 2 lemon juices • 2 tablespoons honey

Directions:

1. Put in water into a deep cooking pan. Put the deep cooking pan on moderate heat.

2. When it starts to boil, put in turmeric, cinnamon, and ginger and stir slowly.

3. Remove the heat. Cover and allow the mixture to steep for 12–fifteen minutes. Put in honey and lemon juice.

4. Stir and pour into mugs.

5. Serve.

Nutritional Info: Calories: 121 kcal , Protein: 3.57 g , Fat: 3.2 g , Carbohydrates: 21.97 g

8. VANILLA AVOCADO SMOOTHIE

Time To Prepare: ten minutes

Time to Cook: 0 minutes **Yield:** Servings 1

Ingredients:

- 1 cup almond milk

- 1 ripe avocado, halved and pitted

- 1/2 cup vanilla yogurt

- 3 tbsp. honey

- 8 ice cubes

Directions:

1. Put in everything to a blender jug.

2. Cover the jug firmly.

3. Blend until the desired smoothness is achieved. Serve and enjoy!

Nutritional Info: Calories: 143 , Fat: 1.2 g , Protein: 4.6 g , Carbohydrates: 21 g , Fiber: 2.3 g

9. VANILLA BLUEBERRY SMOOTHIE

Time To Prepare: five minutes

Time to Cook: 0 minutes **Yield:** Servings 1

Ingredients:

- cup fresh blueberries

- tbsp. flaxseed oil

- cups hemp milk

- 2 tbsp. hemp protein powder

- Handful of ice/ 1 cup frozen blueberries

Directions:

1. Mix milk and fresh blueberries plus ice (or frozen blueberries) in a blender.

2. Blend for a minute, move to a glass, and mix in flaxseed oil.

Nutritional Info: Calories: 1041 kcal , Protein: 35.21 g , Fat: 41.04 g , Carbohydrates: 140.4 g

10. VANILLA TURMERIC ORANGE JUICE

Time To Prepare: five minutes

Time to Cook: 0 minutes **Yield:** Servings 2

Ingredients:

- ½ teaspoon turmeric powder

- 1 teaspoon ground cinnamon

- 2 cups unsweetened almond milk

- 2 teaspoons vanilla extract

- 6 oranges, peeled, separated into segments, deseeded

- Pepper to taste

Directions:

1. Juice the oranges. Put in the remaining ingredients.

2. Pour into 2 glasses before you serve.

Nutritional Info: Calories: 223 kcal , Protein: 11.47 g , Fat: 11.79 g , Carbohydrates: fifteen.9 g

11.   VOLUPTUOUS VANILLA HOT DRINK

Time To Prepare: ten minutes

Time to Cook: 0 minutes **Yield:** Servings 1

Ingredients:

- 1 scoop of hemp protein

- 1/2 Tbsp. ground cinnamon (or more to taste)

- 1/2 Tbsp. vanilla extract

- 3 cups unsweetened almond milk (or 1 1/2 cup full-fat coconut milk + 1 1/2 cups water) • Stevia to taste

Directions:

1.   Put the almond milk into a pitcher. Put ground cinnamon, hemp, vanilla extract in a small deep cooking pan on moderate to high heat. Heat until the pure liquid stevia is just melted and then pour the pure liquid stevia mixture into the pitcher.

2.   Stir until the pure liquid stevia is well blended with the almond milk. Bring the pitcher in your refrigerator and let it cool for minimum two hours. Stir thoroughly before you serve.

Nutritional Info: Calories: 656 kcal , Protein: 42.12 g , Fat: 33.05 g , Carbohydrates: 44.45 g

12.   WASSAIL

Time To Prepare: five minutes

Time to Cook: ten minutes **Yield:** Servings 4

Ingredients:

• • ½ tsp nutmeg

• inch peeled ginger

• 10 cloves

• 2 vanilla beans, split or 2 Tbsp pure vanilla extract

• cups orange juice

• cinnamon sticks

• • 8 cups apple cider • Zest and juice of 2 lemons

Directions:

1. Pour cider and orange juice in the instant pot.

2. Put cinnamon sticks, nutmeg piece, cloves, lemon zest, vanilla beans in the steamer basket.

3. If you didn't use vanilla beans, pour in vanilla extract. Put in lemon juice.

4. Secure the lid. Cook on HIGH pressure ten minutes.

5. When done, depressurize naturally.

6. Discard contents of the steamer basket.

7. Serve hot from the pot.

Nutritional Info: Calories: 221 , Fat: 0g , Carbohydrates: 42g , Protein: 0g

13.   WHITE HOT CHOCOLATE

Time To Prepare: five minutes

Time to Cook: six minutes **Yield:** Servings 2

Ingredients:

- ¼ cup cocoa powder/butter

- 2 - 2½ Tbsp honey

- 2 tsp vanilla extract

- 3 cups coconut milk

- Pinch of sea salt

Directions:

1. Put in milk, cocoa powder/butter, honey, vanilla extract, and salt to the instant pot.

2. Secure the lid. Cook on LOW pressure six minutes.

3. Depressurize swiftly.

4. Use a hand blender to blend contents 25 seconds.

5. Serve hot.

Nutritional Info: Calories: 331 , Fat: 14g , Carbohydrates: 47g , Protein: 4g

14. WONDERFUL WATERMELON DRINK

Time To Prepare: five minutes

Time to Cook: 0 minutes **Yield:** Servings 2

Ingredients:

- 1 cup of coconut water

- 1 cup of watermelon chunks

- 1/2 cup of tart cherries

- 2 cups of frozen mixed berries

- 2 tbsp. of chia seeds

Directions:

1. Combine all ingredients in a blender or juicer then blend until pureed.

2. Serve instantly and enjoy!

Nutritional Info: Calories: 330 kcal , Protein: 10.22 g , Fat: 9.71 g , Carbohydrates: 53.3 g

15.   ZESTY CITRUS SMOOTHIE

Time To Prepare: five minutes

Time to Cook: 0 minutes **Yield:** Servings 1

Ingredients:

• cup almond milk

• 1 med orange peeled, cleaned, and cut into sections

• 1 tbsp. flaxseed oil 2 tsp hemp protein powder half cup lemon juice

• • Handful of ice

Directions:

1. Mix milk, lemon juice, orange, and ice in a blender.

2. Blend for a minute, move to a glass, and mix in flaxseed oil.

Nutritional Info: Calories: 427 kcal , Protein: 17.5 g , Fat: 28.88 g , Carbohydrates: 24.96 g

16.   BEET HUMMUS

Time To Prepare: five minutes

Time to Cook: 0 minutes **Yield:** Servings 2

Ingredients:

- ¼ tsp of chili flakes ½ cup of olive oil

- ½ tsp of oregano • ½ tsp of salt

- 1 ½ tsp of cumin 1 ¾ cup of chickpeas

- 1 clove of garlic

- 1 nub of fresh ginger

- 1 skinless roasted beet

- 1 tsp of curry

- 1 tsp of maple syrup

- 2 tbsp. of sunflower seeds

- Juice of one lemon

Directions:

1. Blend all together the ingredients in a food processor until they're smooth and decorate them with sunflower seeds.

2. Enjoy!

Nutritional Info: , Calories: 423 kcal , Protein: 13.98 g , Fat: 24.26 g , Carbohydrates: 40.13 g

17.   BROCCOLI AND BLACK BEANS STIR FRY

Time To Prepare: ten minutes

Time to Cook: fifteen minutes **Yield:** Servings 4

Ingredients:

- 1 tablespoon sesame oil

- 2 cloves garlic, thoroughly minced

- 2 cups cooked black beans

- 2 teaspoons ginger, finely chopped

- 4 cups broccoli florets

- 4 teaspoons sesame seeds

- A big pinch red chili flakes

- A pinch turmeric powder

- Lime juice to taste (not necessary)

- Salt to taste

Directions:

1. Pour enough water to immerse the bottom of the deep cooking pan by an inch. Put a strainer on the deep cooking pan. Put broccoli florets on the strainer. Steam the broccoli for about six minutes.

2. Put a big frying pan on moderate heat. Put in sesame oil. When the oil is just warm, put in sesame seeds, chili flakes, ginger, garlic, turmeric powder and salt. Sauté for about 2 minutes until aromatic.

3. Put in steamed broccoli and black beans and sauté until meticulously heated.

4. Put in lime juice and stir.

5. Serve hot.

Nutritional Info: , Calories: 196 kcal , Protein: 11.2 g , Fat: 7.25 g , Carbohydrates: 23.45 g

18.   CARAMELIZED PEARS AND ONIONS

Time To Prepare: five minutes

Time to Cook: thirty-five minutes **Yield:** Servings 4

Ingredients:

- 1 tablespoon olive oil

- 2 firm red pears, cored and quartered

- 2 red onion, cut into wedges

- Salt and pepper, to taste

Directions:

1. Preheat the oven to 425 degrees F

2. Put the pears and onion on a baking tray

3. Sprinkle with olive oil

4. Sprinkle with salt and pepper

5. Bake using your oven for a little more than half an hour

6. Serve and enjoy!

Nutritional Info: , Calories: 101 , Fat: 4g , Carbohydrates: 17g , Protein: 1g

19. CAULIFLOWER BROCCOLI MASH

Time To Prepare: five minutes

Time to Cook: ten minutes **Yield:** Servings 6

Ingredients:

- 1 big head cauliflower, cut into chunks

- 1 small head broccoli, cut into florets

- 1 teaspoon salt

- 3 tablespoons extra virgin olive oil

- Pepper, to taste

Directions:

1. Take a pot and put in oil then heat it

2. Put in the cauliflower and broccoli

3. Sprinkle with salt and pepper to taste

4. Keep stirring to make vegetable soft

5. Put in water if required

6. When is already cooked, use a food processor or a potato masher to puree the vegetables

7. Serve and enjoy!

Nutritional Info: , Calories: 39 , Fat: 3g , Carbohydrates: 2g , Protein: 0.89g

20. CILANTRO AND AVOCADO PLATTER

Time To Prepare: ten minutes

Time to Cook: 0 minutes **Yield:** Servings 6

Ingredients:

- ¼ cup of fresh cilantro, chopped

- ½ a lime, juiced

- 1 big ripe tomato, chopped

- 1 green bell pepper, chopped

- 1 sweet onion, chopped

- 2 avocados, peeled, pitted and diced

- Salt and pepper as required

Directions:

1. Take a moderate-sized container and put in onion, bell pepper, tomato, avocados, lime and cilantro

2. Mix thoroughly and give it a toss

3. Sprinkle with salt and pepper in accordance with your taste

4. Serve and enjoy!

Nutritional Info: , Calories: 126 , Fat: 10g , Carbohydrates: 10g , Protein: 2g

21. CITRUS COUSCOUS WITH HERB

Time To Prepare: five minutes

Time to Cook: fifteen minutes **Yield:** Servings 2

Ingredients:

- ¼ cup of water

- ¼ orange, chopped

- ½ teaspoon butter

- 1 teaspoon Italian seasonings

- 1/3 cup couscous

- 1/3 teaspoon salt

- 4 tablespoons orange juice

Directions:

1. Pour water and orange juice in the pan.

2. Put in orange, Italian seasoning, and salt.

3. Bring the liquid to boil and take it off the heat.

4. Put in butter and couscous. Stir thoroughly and close the lid.

5. Leave the couscous rest for about ten minutes.

Nutritional Info: Calories 149 , Fat: 1.9 , Fiber: 2.1 , Carbs: 28.5 , Protein: 4.1

22. COOL GARBANZO AND SPINACH BEANS

Time To Prepare: 5-ten minutes

Time to Cook: 0 minute **Yield:** Servings 4

Ingredients:

- ½ onion, diced

- ½ teaspoon cumin

- 1 tablespoon olive oil

- 10 ounces spinach, chopped

- 12 ounces garbanzo beans

Directions:

1. Take a frying pan and put in olive oil

2. Put it on moderate to low heat

3. Put in onions, garbanzo and cook for five minutes

4. Mix in cumin, garbanzo beans, spinach and flavor with sunflower seeds

5. Use a spoon to smash gently 6. Cook meticulously

7. Serve and enjoy!

Nutritional Info: , Calories: 90 , Fat: 4g , Carbohydrates:11g , Protein:4g

23.   COUSCOUS SALAD

Time To Prepare: ten minutes

Time to Cook: six minutes

Yield: Servings 4

Ingredients:

- ¼ teaspoon ground black pepper

- ¾ teaspoon ground coriander

- ½ teaspoon salt

- ¼ teaspoon paprika

- ¼ teaspoon turmeric

- 1 tablespoon butter

- 2 oz. chickpeas, canned, drained

- 1 cup fresh arugula, chopped

- 2 oz. sun-dried tomatoes, chopped

- 1 oz. Feta cheese, crumbled

- 1 tablespoon canola oil

- 1/3 cup couscous • 1/3 cup chicken stock

Directions:

1. Bring the chicken stock to boil.

2. Put in couscous, ground black pepper, ground coriander, salt, paprika, and turmeric. Put in chickpeas and butter. Mix the mixture well and close the lid.

3. Allow the couscous soak the hot chicken stock for about six minutes.

4. In the meantime, in the mixing container mix together arugula, sun-dried tomatoes, and Feta cheese.

5. Put in cooked couscous mixture and canola oil.

6. Mix up the salad well.

Nutritional Info: Calories 18 , Fat: 9 , Fiber: 3.6 , Carbs: 21.1 , Protein: 6

24.   CREAMY POLENTA

Time To Prepare: 8 minutes

Time to Cook: forty-five minutes **Yield:** Servings 4

Ingredients:

- ½ cup cream

- 1 ½ cup water

- 1 cup polenta

- 1/3 cup Parmesan, grated

- 2 cups chicken stock

Directions:

1. Put polenta in the pot.

2. Put in water, chicken stock, cream, and Parmesan. Mix up polenta well.

3. Then preheat oven to 355F.

4. Cook polenta in your oven for about forty-five minutes.

5. Mix up the cooked meal with the help of the spoon cautiously before you serve.

Nutritional Info: Calories 208 , Fat: 5.3 , Fiber: 1 , Carbs: 32.2 , Protein: 8

25.   CRISPY CORN

Time To Prepare: 8 minutes

Time to Cook: five minutes **Yield:** Servings 3

Ingredients:

- ½ teaspoon ground paprika ½ teaspoon salt

- ¾ teaspoon chili pepper

- 1 cup corn kernels

- 1 tablespoon coconut flour

- 1 tablespoon water • 3 tablespoons canola oil

Directions:

1. In the mixing container, mix together corn kernels with salt and coconut flour.

2. Put in water and mix up the corn with the help of the spoon.

3. Pour canola oil in the frying pan and heat it.

4. Put in corn kernels mixture and roast it for about four minutes. Stir it occasionally.

5. When the corn kernels are crispy, move them in the plate and dry with the paper towel's help.

6. Put in chili pepper and ground paprika. Mix up well.

Nutritional Info: Calories 179 , Fat: fifteen , Fiber: 2.4 , Carbs: 11.3 , Protein: 2.1

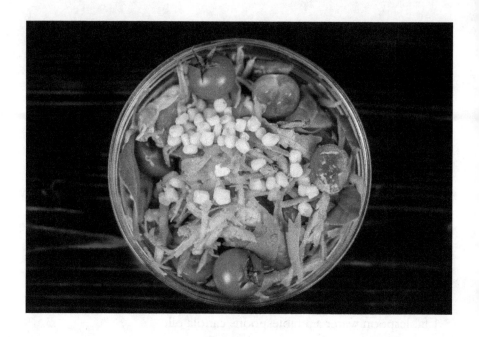

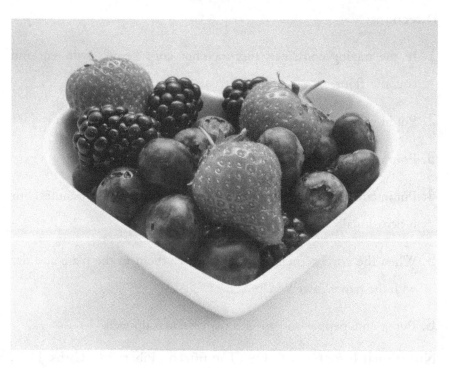

26. CUCUMBER YOGURT SALAD WITH MINT

Time To Prepare: ten minutes

Time to Cook: 0 minutes **Yield:** Servings 2

Ingredients:

- ¼ cup organic coconut milk

- ¼ cup organic mint leaves

- ¼ teaspoon pink Himalayan sea salt

- ½ cup chopped organic red onion

- 1 tablespoon extra virgin olive oil

- 1 tablespoon plain organic goat yogurt

- 1 teaspoon organic dill weed

- 2 chopped organic cucumbers • 3 tablespoons fresh organic lime juice

Directions:

1. Cut the red onion, dill, cucumbers, and mint and mix them in a big container.

2. Blend them until they're smooth. Top the dressing onto the cucumber salad and mix meticulously. Chill for minimum 1 hour and serve.

Nutritional Info: , Calories: 207 kcal , Protein: 6.9 g , Fat: 13.87 g , Carbohydrates: 18.04 g

27.   CURRY WHEATBERRY RICE

Time To Prepare: ten minutes

Time to Cook: 1 hour fifteen minutes **Yield:** Servings 5

Ingredients:

- ¼ cup milk

- ½ cup of rice

- 1 cup wheat berries

- 1 tablespoon curry paste

- 1 teaspoon salt

- 4 tablespoons olive oil

- 6 cups chicken stock

Directions:

1. Put wheatberries and chicken stock in the pan.

2. Close the lid and cook the mixture for an hour over the moderate heat.

3. Then put in rice, olive oil, and salt.

4. Stir thoroughly.

5. Mix up together milk and curry paste.

6. Put in the curry liquid in the rice-wheatberry mixture and stir thoroughly.

7. Boil the meal for fifteen minutes with the closed lid.

8. When the rice is cooked, all the meal is cooked.

Nutritional Info: Calories 232 , Fat: fifteen , Fiber: 1.4 , Carbs: 23.5 ,
Protein: 3.9

28.   FARRO SALAD WITH ARUGULA

Time To Prepare: ten minutes

Time to Cook: thirty-five minutes **Yield:** Servings 2

Ingredients:

- ½ cup farro

- ½ teaspoon ground black pepper

- ½ teaspoon Italian seasoning

- ½ teaspoon olive oil

- 1 ½ cup chicken stock

- 1 cucumber, chopped

- 1 tablespoon lemon juice

- 1 teaspoon salt • 2 cups arugula, chopped

Directions:

1. Mix up together farro, salt, and chicken stock and move mixture in the pan.

2. Close the lid and boil it for a little more than half an hour.

3. In the meantime, place all rest of the ingredients in the salad container.

4. Chill the farro to the room temperature and put in it in the salad container too.

5. Mix up the salad well.

Nutritional Info: Calories 92 , Fat: 2.3 , Fiber: 2 , Carbs: 15.6 , Protein: 3.9

29.   FETA CHEESE SALAD

Time To Prepare: ten minutes

Time to Cook: 0 minutes **Yield:** Servings 2

Ingredients:

- 1 tbsp. olive oil (extra virgin)

- 1 tsp balsamic vinegar

- 2 cucumbers

- 30 g feta cheese

- 4 spring onions

- 4 tomatoes Salt

Directions:

1. Cube the tomatoes and cucumbers.

2. Thinly slice the onions.

3. Crush the feta cheese.

4. Mix tomatoes, onions, and cucumbers.

5. Put olive oil, vinegar, and a small amount of salt.

6. Put in feta cheese.

7. Enjoy your meal!

Nutritional Info: , Calories: 221 kcal , Protein: 9.24 g , Fat: 13.84 g , Carbohydrates: 17.18 g

30.   FRESH STRAWBERRY SALSA

Time To Prepare: ten minutes

Time to Cook: 0 minutes **Yield:** Servings 6-8

Ingredients:

- ¼ cup fresh lime juice

- ½ cup fresh cilantro

- ½ cup red onion, finely chopped

- ½ teaspoon lime zest, grated

- 1-2 jalapeños, deseeded, finely chopped

- 2 kiwi fruit, peeled, chopped

- 2 pounds fresh ripe strawberries, hulled, chopped

- 2 teaspoons pure raw honey

Directions:

1. Put in lime juice, lime zest and honey into a big container and whisk well.

2. Put in remaining ingredients then mix thoroughly.

3. Cover and set aside for a while for the flavors to set in and serve.

Nutritional Info: , Calories: 119 kcal , Protein: 9.26 g , Fat: 4.38 g , Carbohydrates: 11.73 g

31.   GOAT CHEESE SALAD

Time To Prepare: fifteen minutes

Time to Cook: thirty minutes **Yield:** Servings 4

Ingredients:

- ½ cup of walnuts

- ½ head of escarole (medium), torn

- 1 bunch of trimmed and torn arugula

- 1/3 cup extra virgin olive oil

- 2 bunches of medium beets (~1 ½ lbs.) with trimmed tops

- 2 tbsp. of red wine vinegar

- 4 oz. crumbled of goat cheese (aged cheese is preferred)

- Kosher salt + freshly ground black pepper

Directions:

1. Place the beets in water in a deep cooking pan and apply salt as seasoning. Now, boil them using high heat for approximately twenty minutes or until they're soft. Peel them off when they're cool using your fingers or use a knife.

2. To taste, whisk the vinegar with salt and pepper in a big container. Then mix in the olive oil for the dressing. Toss the beets with the dressing, so they're uniformly coated and marinate them for approximately fifteen minutes– 2 hours.

3. Set the oven to 350F. Bring the nuts on a baking sheet and toast them for approximately 8 minutes (stirring them once) until they turn golden brown.

Let them cool.

4. Mix and toss the escarole and arugula with the beets and put them in four plates. Put in the walnuts and goat cheese as toppings before you serve.

5. Enjoy!

Nutritional Info: , Calories: 285 kcal , Protein: 11.85 g , Fat: 25.79 g , Carbohydrates: 2.01 g

32.   GREEN BEANS

Time To Prepare: five minutes

Time to Cook: ten minutes **Yield:** Servings 5

Ingredients:

- ½ teaspoon kosher salt

- ½ teaspoon of red pepper flakes

- 1½ lbs. green beans, trimmed

- 2 garlic cloves, minced

- 2 tablespoons of extra-virgin olive oil

- 2 tablespoons of water

Directions:

1. Heat oil in a frying pan on medium temperature.

2. Include the pepper flake. Stir to coat in the olive oil.

3. Include the green beans. Cook for seven minutes.

4. Stir frequently. The beans must be brown in some areas.

5. Put in the salt and garlic. Cook for a minute, while stirring.

6. Pour water and cover instantly.

7. Cook covered for 1 more minute.

Nutritional Info: Calories 82 , Carbohydrates: 6g , Total Fat: 6g , Protein: 1g , Fiber: 2g , Sugar: 0g , Sodium: 230mg

33.   GREEN, RED AND YELLOW RICE

Time To Prepare: five minutes

Time to Cook: fifteen minutes

Yield: Servings 10

Ingredients:

• ¼ cup garlic, finely chopped

• 1 cup fresh cilantro, chopped

• 2 cups brown rice, washed

• 2 cups frozen corn, thawed

• 2 cups green onions, chopped

• 2 cups red bell pepper, chopped

• 2 tablespoons olive oil

• Cayenne pepper to taste

• Pepper to taste

• Salt to taste

Directions:

1. Put a big deep cooking pan on moderate heat. Put in 4 cups water and brown rice and cook in accordance with the instructions on the package.

Once cooked, cover and save for later.

2. Put a big frying pan on moderate heat. Put in oil. When the oil is heated, put in garlic and sauté for approximately one minute until aromatic.

3. Put in corn, red bell pepper, green onion, salt, pepper and cayenne pepper and sauté for at least two minutes.

4. Put in rice and cilantro. Mix thoroughly and heat meticulously.

5. Serve.

Nutritional Info: , Calories: 89 kcal , Protein: 2.41 g , Fat: 4.01 g , Carbohydrates: 11.26 g

34.   HOT PINK COCONUT SLAW

Time To Prepare: five minutes

Time to Cook: 0 minutes **Yield:** Servings 3

Ingredients:

- ¼ cup fresh cilantro, chopped

- ¼ teaspoon salt

- ½ cup big coconut flakes, unsweetened or shredded coconut, unsweetened

- ½ cup radish, thinly cut or shredded carrots

- ½ small jalapeño, deseeded, discard membranes, chopped

- ½ tablespoon honey or maple syrup

- 1 cup red onion, thinly cut

- 1 tablespoon olive oil 2 cups purple cabbage, thinly cut

- 2 tablespoons apple cider vinegar 2 tablespoons lime juice

Directions:

1. Combine all ingredients into a container and toss thoroughly. Cover and set aside for about forty minutes.

2. Toss thoroughly before you serve.

Nutritional Info: , Calories: 179 kcal , Protein: 3.92 g , Fat: 10.64 g , Carbohydrates: 18.53 g

35.   LENTIL SALAD

Time To Prepare: ten minutes

Time to Cook: 0 minutes **Yield:** Servings 2

Ingredients:

- ½ cup parsley

- 1 red bell pepper - 1 tbsp. lime juice - 1 tbsp. olive oil

- 2 cups lentil - 3 spring onions

- A pinch of salt

- fifteen basil leaves

- Turmeric– to your taste

Directions:

1. Cook the lentils based on the package instructions. Put in a garlic clove while cooking.

2. When cooled, remove the garlic clove and put the lentils into a big container.

3. Chop all the vegetables then put in them to the lentils.

4. Put in lime juice, a small amount of salt, and olive oil.

5. Mix thoroughly.

Nutritional Info: , Calories: 207 kcal , Protein: 11.53 g , Fat: 10.49 g , Carbohydrates: 22.37 g

36.   MASCARPONE COUSCOUS

Time To Prepare: fifteen minutes

Time to Cook: 7.5 hours **Yield:** Servings 4

Ingredients:

- ½ cup mascarpone

- 1 cup couscous

- 1 teaspoon ground paprika

- 1 teaspoon salt • 3 ½ cup chicken stock

Directions:

1. Put chicken stock and mascarpone in the pan and bring the liquid to boil.

2. Put in salt and ground paprika. Stir gently and simmer for a minute.

3. Take off the liquid from the heat and put in couscous. Stir thoroughly and close the lid.

4. Leave couscous for about ten minutes.

5. Mix the cooked side dish well before you serve.

Nutritional Info: Calories 227 , Fat: 4.9 , Fiber: 2.4 , Carbs: 35.4 , Protein: 9.7

37.   MOROCCAN STYLE COUSCOUS

Time To Prepare: ten minutes

Time to Cook: ten minutes **Yield:** Servings 4

Ingredients:

- ½ teaspoon ground cardamom

- ½ teaspoon red pepper

- 1 cup chicken stock

- 1 cup yellow couscous

- 1 tablespoon butter

- 1 teaspoon salt

Directions:

1. Toss butter in the pan and melt it.

2. Put in couscous and roast it for a minute over the high heat.

3. Then put in ground cardamom, salt, and red pepper. Stir it well.

4. Pour the chicken stock and bring the mixture to boil.

5. Simmer couscous for five minutes with the closed lid.

Nutritional Info: Calories 196 , Fat: 3.4 , Fiber: 2.4 , Carbs: 35 , Protein: 5.9

38.   MUSHROOM MILLET

Time To Prepare: ten minutes

Time to Cook: fifteen minutes **Yield:** Servings 3

Ingredients:

- ¼ cup mushrooms, cut

- ½ cup millet

- ¾ cup onion, diced

- 1 cup of water

- 1 tablespoon olive oil

- 1 teaspoon butter

- 1 teaspoon salt • 3 tablespoons milk

Directions:

1. Pour olive oil in the frying pan then put the onion.

2. Put in mushrooms and roast the vegetables for about ten minutes over the moderate heat. Stir them occasionally.

3. In the meantime, pour water in the pan.

4. Put in millet and salt.

5. Cook the millet with the closed lid for fifteen minutes over the moderate heat.

6. Then put in the cooked mushroom mixture in the millet.

7. Put in milk and butter. Mix up the millet well.

Nutritional Info: Calories 198 , Fat: 7.7 , Fiber: 3.5 , Carbs: 27.9 , Protein: 4.7

39. ONION AND ORANGE HEALTHY SALAD

Time To Prepare: ten minutes

Time to Cook: 0 minutes **Yield:** Servings 3

Ingredients:

- ¼ cup of fresh chives, chopped

- 1 cup olive oil

- 1 red onion, thinly cut

- 1 teaspoon of dried oregano

- 3 tablespoon of red wine vinegar

- 6 big orange

- 6 tablespoon of olive oil

- Ground black pepper

Directions:

1. Peel the orange and cut each of them in 4-5 crosswise slices

2. Move the oranges to a shallow dish

3. Sprinkle vinegar, olive oil and drizzle oregano

4. Toss

5. Chill for thirty minutes

6. Position cut onion and black olives on top

7. Garnish with an additional drizzle of chives and a fresh grind of pepper

8. Serve and enjoy!

Nutritional Info: , Calories: 120 , Fat: 6g , Carbohydrates: 20g , Protein: 2g

40.   PARMESAN ROASTED BROCCOLI

Time To Prepare: ten minutes **Time to Cook:** twenty minutes **Yield:** Servings 6

Ingredients:

- ½ teaspoon of Italian seasoning

- 1 tablespoon of lemon juice

- 1 tablespoon parsley, chopped

- 3 tablespoons of olive oil

- 3 tablespoons of vegan parmesan, grated

- 4 cups of broccoli florets

- Pepper and salt to taste

Directions:

1. Preheat the oven to 450 degrees F. Apply cooking spray on your pan.

2. Keep the broccoli florets in a freezer bag.

3. Now put in the Italian seasoning, olive oil, pepper, and salt.

4. Seal your bag. Shake it. Coat well.

5. Pour your broccoli on the pan. It must be in a single layer.

6. Bake for about twenty minutes. Stir midway through.

7. Take out from the oven. Drizzle parsley and parmesan. Sprinkle some lemon juice.

8. You can decorate with lemon wedges if you wish.

Nutritional Info: Calories 96 , Carbohydrates: 4g , Cholesterol: 2mg , Total Fat: 8g , Protein: 2g , Sugar: 1g , Fiber: 1g , Sodium: 58mg , Potassium: 191mg

41.   QUINOA SALAD

Time To Prepare: ten minutes

Time to Cook: 0 minutes **Yield:** Servings 2

Ingredients:

- ¼ tsp sea salt

- ½ cup quinoa (uncooked)

- 1 carrot

- 1 tbsp. apple cider vinegar

- 1 tbsp. flaxseed oil

- 2 brussels sprouts

Directions:

1. Wash quinoa meticulously.

2. Dice the carrots and brussels sprouts to minuscule pieces.

3. Cook the quinoa based on the instruction on the packaging. Mix flaxseed oil, sea salt, and apple cider vinegar. Sauté brussels sprouts and carrots on a small amount of olive oil for a few minutes.

4. After both brussels sprouts and carrots, and quinoa are ready, combine them all in a container. Put in the dressing and mix meticulously. Serve warm.

Nutritional Info: , Calories: 280 kcal **,** Protein: 10.15 g **,** Fat: 12.52 g **,** Carbohydrates: 31.99 g

42.   RED CABBAGE WITH CHEESE

Time To Prepare: five minutes

Time to Cook: twelve minutes **Yield:** Servings 4

Ingredients:

- ¼ cup & 1 tbsp. of extra virgin olive oil

- ¼ tsp of freshly ground pepper

- ¼ tsp of salt

- 1 cup of walnuts

- 1 Tbsp. of crumbled blue cheese

- 1 tbsp. of Dijon mustard

- 1 tsp of butter

- 2 thinly cut scallions

- 3 tbsp. of pure maple syrup

- 3 tbsp. of red wine vinegar • 8 cups of red cabbage, thinly cut

Directions:

For the vinaigrette:

1. Combine the blue cheese, ¼ cup of olive oil, mustard, vinegar, salt, and pepper in a food processor or blender until the mixture has a creamy consistency.

For the salad:

1. Put a parchment paper near the stove.

2. Heat 1 tbsp. Of oil on moderate heat in a moderate-sized frying pan and mix in the walnuts, cooking them for approximately 2 minutes. 3. Now mix salt and pepper, sprinkle maple syrup and cook for approximately three to five minutes while stirring the mixture up to the nuts are uniformly coated.

4. Move to the paper and pour the rest of the syrup over them using a spoon. Separate the nuts and cool down for approximately five minutes.

5. In a big container, put in the cabbage and scallions and toss them with the vinaigrette. Put in the walnuts and blue cheese as toppings.

Nutritional Info: Calories 232 , Fat: 19 gram Saturated , Fat: 4 gram , Sodium: 267 gram , Carbs: 12 gram , Fiber: 2 gram sugar , 8 gram Added sugar 5 gram , Protein: 4 gram

43.   RICE WITH PISTACHIOS

Time To Prepare: ten minutes **Time to Cook:** twenty minutes **Yield:**
Servings 6

Ingredients:

- ¼ cup of raw pistachios (or more for decoration)

- ½ cup of chopped and packed dill leaves

- ½ teaspoon of turmeric

- 1 ½ cups of Basmati rice (rinsed in a colander and soaked in water for
  approximately 30 minutes, or

more)

- 1 teaspoon of vegetable oil

- 1 thinly cut medium onion

- 2 dry baby leaves

- 3 cups of vegetable stock or water

- 5 pods of slightly crushed green cardamom

- Ground black pepper (to taste)

- Salt, to taste

Directions:

1. In a big deep cooking pan, warm the oil and put in the cardamom. Heat it for approximately 1 minute until it turns smildly brown and put in the onion.

Sauté for approximately 1-2 minutes.

2. Mix in the dill leaves, turmeric and pistachios. Then put in the rice and stir-fry for approximately one minute.

3. Combine the vegetable stock, black pepper and salt to taste, stir it well and bring it to its boiling point.

4. Cover the pan using lid and cook on moderate to low heat for approximately fifteen minutes.

5. Take it off from the heat then set aside the rice (covered) for approximately ten minutes. Then fluff it using a fork and put in more pistachios as decorate, if you desire.

6. Enjoy!

Nutritional Info: , Calories: 90 kcal , Protein: 3.36 g , Fat: 5.08 g , Carbohydrates: 8.39 g

44. ROASTED CARROTS

Time To Prepare: ten minutes

Time to Cook: forty minutes **Yield:** Servings 4

Ingredients:

- ¼ teaspoon ground pepper

- ½ teaspoon rosemary, chopped

- ½ teaspoon salt

- 1 onion, peeled & cut

- 1 teaspoon thyme, chopped

- 2 tablespoons of extra-virgin olive oil

- 8 carrots, peeled & cut

Directions:

1. Preheat the oven to 425 degrees F.

2. Combine the onions and carrots by tossing in a container with rosemary, thyme, pepper, and salt. Spread on your baking sheet.

3. Roast for forty minutes. The onions and carrots must be browning and soft.

Nutritional Info: Calories 126 , Carbohydrates: 16g , Total Fat: 6g , Protein: 2g , Fiber: 4g , Sugar: 8g , Sodium: 286mg

45.　　ROASTED CURRIED CAULIFLOWER

Time To Prepare: five minutes

Time to Cook: thirty minutes **Yield:** Servings 4

Ingredients:

- ¾ teaspoon salt

- 1 and ½ tablespoon olive oil

- 1 big head cauliflower, cut into florets

- 1 teaspoon cumin seeds

- 1 teaspoon curry powder • 1 teaspoon mustard seeds

Directions:

1. Preheat the oven to 375 degrees F

2. Grease a baking sheet with cooking spray

3. Take a container and place all ingredients

4. Toss to coat well

5. Position the vegetable on a baking sheet 6. Roast for thirty minutes

7. Serve and enjoy!

Nutritional Info: , Calories: 67 , Fat: 6g , Carbohydrates: 4g , Protein: 2g

46.   ROASTED PARSNIPS

Time To Prepare: five minutes

Time to Cook: thirty minutes **Yield:** Servings 4

Ingredients:

- 1 tablespoon of extra-virgin olive oil

- 1 teaspoon of kosher salt

- 1½ teaspoon of Italian seasoning

- 2 lbs. parsnips

- Chopped parsley for decoration

Directions:

1. Preheat the oven to 400 degrees F.

2. Peel the parsnips. Cut them into one-inch chunks.

3. Now toss with the seasoning, salt, and oil in a container.

4. Spread this on your baking sheet. It must be in a single layer.

5. Roast for half an hour Stir every ten minutes.

6. Move to a plate. Decorate using parsley.

Nutritional Info: Calories 124 , Carbohydrates: 20g , Total Fat: 4g , Protein: 2g , Fiber: 4g , Sugar: 5g , Sodium: 550mg

47. ROASTED PORTOBELLOS WITH ROSEMARY

Time To Prepare: five minutes

Time to Cook: fifteen minutes **Yield:** Servings 4

Ingredients:

- ¼ cup extra virgin olive oil

- 1 clove garlic, minced

- 1 sprig rosemary, torn

- 2 tablespoons fresh lemon juice

- 8 portobello mushroom, trimmed

- Salt and pepper, to taste

Directions:

1. Preheat the oven to 450 degrees F

2. Take a container and put in all ingredients

3. Toss to coat

4. Put the mushroom in a baking sheet stem side up

5. Roast in your oven for fifteen minutes

6. Serve and enjoy!

Nutritional Info: , Calories: 63 , Fat: 6g , Carbohydrates: 2g , Protein:1g

48.   SHOEPEG CORN SALAD

Time To Prepare: ten minutes

Time to Cook: 0 minute **Yield:** Servings 4

Ingredients:

- ¼ cup Greek yogurt

- ½ cup cherry tomatoes halved

- 1 cup shoepeg corn, drained

- 1 jalapeno pepper, chopped

- 1 tablespoon chives, chopped

- 1 tablespoon lemon juice

- 3 tablespoons fresh cilantro, chopped

Directions:

1. In the salad container, mix up together shoepeg corn, cherry tomatoes, jalapeno pepper, chives, and fresh cilantro.

2. Put in lemon juice and Greek yogurt. Mix yo the salad well.

3. Put in your fridge and store it for maximum 1 day.

Nutritional Info: Calories 49 , Fat: 0.7 , Fiber: 1.2 , Carbs: 9.4 , Protein: 2.7

49.   SPICED SWEET POTATO BREAD

Time To Prepare: fifteen minutes

Time to Cook: 45-55 minutes

Yield: Servings 2

Ingredients:

For dry Ingredients :

- ¼ teaspoon sea salt

- 1 cup coconut flour

- 1 teaspoon ground mace

- 2 tablespoons ground cinnamon

- 2 teaspoons baking powder

- 2 teaspoons baking soda • 2 teaspoons ground nutmeg

Wet Ingredients:

- 1 cup almond butter

- 2 teaspoons organic almond extract

- 4 big sweet potatoes, peeled, thinly cut

- 4 tablespoons coconut oil

- 8 big eggs

- 8 tablespoons melted grass fed butter, unsalted

Directions:

1. Grease 2 loaf pans of 9 x 5 inches with coconut oil. Coat the bottom of the pan using parchment paper. Set aside.

2. Put a medium deep cooking pan on moderate heat. Put in sweet potatoes. Pour enough water to immerse the sweet potatoes. Cook until the sweet potatoes are soft.

3. Remove the heat and drain the sweet potatoes.

4. Put in the sweet potatoes back into the pan. Mash with a potato masher until the desired smoothness is achieved. Allow it to cool completely. 5. Put all together the dry ingredients into a container and mix thoroughly. 6. Put in eggs into a big container and whisk well. Put in sweet potatoes, butter, almond extract and almond butter and whisk until well blended.

7. Put in the dry ingredients into the container of wet ingredients and whisk until well blended.

8. Split the batter into the prepared loaf pans.

9. Bake in a preheated oven at 350°F for approximately 45 -55 minutes or a toothpick when inserted in the middle of the loaf comes out clean.

10. Remove from oven and cool to room temperature.

11. Slice using a sharp knife into slices of 1-inch thickness.

Nutritional Info: , Calories: 1738 kcal , Protein: 27 g , Fat: 145.92 g , Carbohydrates: 89.58 g

50. SPICY BARLEY

Time To Prepare: seven minutes

Time to Cook: 42 minutes **Yield:** Servings 5

Ingredients:

- ½ teaspoon cayenne pepper

- ½ teaspoon chili pepper

- ½ teaspoon ground black pepper

- 1 cup barley 1 teaspoon butter

- 1 teaspoon olive oil

- 1 teaspoon salt • 3 cups chicken stock

Directions:

1. Put barley and olive oil in the pan.

2. Roast barley on high heat for a minute. Stir it well.

3. Then put in salt, chili pepper, ground black pepper, cayenne pepper, and butter.

4. Put in chicken stock.

5. Close the lid and cook barley for forty minutes over the medium-low heat.

   Nutritional Info: Calories 152 , Fat: 2.9 , Fiber: 6.5 , Carbs: 27.8 , Protein:5.1

51. SPICY ROASTED BRUSSELS SPROUTS

Time To Prepare: five minutes

Time to Cook: thirty minutes **Yield:** Servings 4

Ingredients:

- ½ cup kimchi with juice

- 1 and ¼ pound Brussels sprouts, cut into florets

- 2 tablespoons olive oil • Salt and pepper, to taste

Directions:

1. Set the oven to 425 F.

2. Toss the Brussels sprouts with pepper, salt, and oil.

3. Bake using your oven for about twenty-five minutes

4. Remove from oven and mix with kimchi. Return to the oven . Cook for five minutes 7. Serve and enjoy!

Nutritional Info: , Calories: 135 , Fat: 7g , Carbohydrates: 16g , Protein: 5g

52.   SPICY WASABI MAYONNAISE

Time To Prepare: fifteen minutes

Time to Cook: 0 minute **Yield:** Servings 4

Ingredients:

- ½ tablespoon wasabi paste

- 1 cup mayonnaise

Directions:

1. Take a container and mix wasabi paste and mayonnaise
Mix thoroughly

2. Allow it to chill, use as required. Serve and enjoy

Nutritional Info: , Calories: 388 , Fat: 42g , Carbohydrates: 1g , Protein: 1g

53.   STIR-FRIED ALMOND AND SPINACH

Time To Prepare: ten minutes

Time to Cook: fifteen minutes **Yield:** Servings 2

Ingredients:

• 1 tablespoon coconut oil

• 3 tablespoons almonds

• 34 pounds spinach

• Salt to taste

Directions:

1. Put oil to a big pot and place it on high heat

2. Put in spinach and allow it to cook, stirring regularly

3. Once the spinach is cooked and soft, sprinkle with salt and stir

4. Put in almonds and enjoy!

Nutritional Info: , Calories: 150 , Fat: 12g , Carbohydrates: 10g , Protein: 8g

54.   STIR-FRIED FARROS

Time To Prepare: five minutes

Time to Cook: thirty-five minutes **Yield:** Servings 2

Ingredients:

- ½ cup farro

- ½ teaspoon ground coriander

- ½ teaspoon paprika

- ½ teaspoon turmeric

- 1 ½ cup water

- 1 carrot, grated

- 1 tablespoon butter

- 1 teaspoon chili flakes

- 1 teaspoon salt • 1 yellow onion, cut

Directions:

1. Put farro in the pan. Put in water and salt.

2. Close the lid and boil it for half an hour

3. In the meantime, toss the butter in the frying pan.

4. Heat it and put in cut onion and grated carrot.

5. Fry the vegetables for about ten minutes over the moderate heat. Stir them with the help of spatula occasionally.

6. When the farro is cooked, put in it in the roasted vegetables and mix up well.

7. Cook stir-fried farro for five minutes over the moderate to high heat.

Nutritional Info: Calories 129 , Fat: 5.9 , Fiber: 3 , Carbs: 17.1 , Protein: 2.8

55.   TENDER FARRO

Time To Prepare: 8 minutes

Time to Cook: forty minutes **Yield:** Servings 4

Ingredients:

- 1 cup farro

- 1 tablespoon almond butter

- 1 tablespoon dried dill

- 1 teaspoon salt • 3 cups beef broth

Directions:

1. Put farro in the pan.

2. Put in beef broth, dried dill, and salt.

3. Close the lid and put the mixture to boil.

4. Then boil it for a little more than half an hour over the medium-low heat.

5. When the time is done, open the lid and put in almond butter.

6. Mix up the cooked farro well.

Nutritional Info: Calories 95 , Fat: 3.3 , Fiber: 1.3 , Carbs: 10.1 , Protein: 6.4

56. THYME WITH HONEY-ROASTED CARROTS

Time To Prepare: five minutes

Time to Cook: thirty minutes **Yield:** Servings 4

Ingredients:

- ½ teaspoon of sea salt

- ½ teaspoon thyme, dried

- 1 tablespoon of honey

- 1/5 lb. carrots, with the tops

- 2 tablespoons of olive oil

Directions:

1. Preheat the oven to 425 degrees F.

2. Place parchment paper on your baking sheet.

3. Toss your carrots with honey, oil, thyme, and salt. Coat well. 4. Keep in a single layer. Bake in the oven for half an hour

5. Allow to cool before you serve.

Nutritional Info: Calories 85 , Carbohydrates: 6g , Cholesterol: 0mg , Total Fat: 8g , Protein: 1g , Sugar: 6g , Fiber: 1g , Sodium: 244mg

57.   TOMATO BULGUR

Time To Prepare: seven minutes

Time to Cook: twenty minutes **Yield:** Servings 2

Ingredients:

- ½ cup bulgur

- ½ white onion, diced

- 1 ½ cup chicken stock

- 1 teaspoon tomato paste • 2 tablespoons coconut oil

Directions:

1. Toss coconut oil in the pan and melt it.

2. Put in diced onion and roast it until light brown.

3. Then put in bulgur and stir thoroughly.

4. Cook bulgur in coconut oil for about three minutes.

5. Then put in tomato paste and mix up bulgur until homogenous.

6. Put in chicken stock.

7. Close the lid and cook bulgur for fifteen minutes over the moderate heat.

8. The cooked bulgur should soak all liquid.

Nutritional Info: Calories 257 , Fat: 14.5 , Fiber: 7.1 , Carbs: 30.2 , Protein: 5.2

58.   WHEATBERRY SALAD

Time To Prepare: ten minutes

Time to Cook: 50 minutes **Yield:** Servings 2

Ingredients:

• ¼ cup fresh parsley, chopped

• ¼ cup of wheat berries

• 1 cup of water 1 tablespoon canola oil

• 1 tablespoon chives, chopped

• 1 teaspoon chili flakes 1 teaspoon salt

• 2 oz. pomegranate seeds • 2 tablespoons walnuts, chopped

Directions:

1. Put wheat berries and water in the pan.

2. Put in salt and simmer the ingredients for about fifty minutes over the moderate heat.

3. In the meantime, mix up together walnuts, chives, parsley, pomegranate seeds, and chili flakes.

4. When the wheatberry is cooked, move it in the walnut mixture.

5. Put in canola oil and mix up the salad well.

Nutritional Info: Calories 160 , Fat: 11.8 , Fiber: 1.2 , Carbs: 12 , Protein: 3.4

59. APPLE AND TOMATO DIPPING SAUCE

Time To Prepare: ten minutes

Time to Cook: 0 minutes **Yield:** Servings 2-4

Ingredients:

- ¼ cup of cider vinegar

- ¼ tsp of freshly ground black pepper

- ½ tsp of sea salt

- 1 garlic clove, finely chopped

- 1 large-sized shallot, diced

- 1 tbsp. natural tomato paste

- 1 tbsp. of extra-virgin olive oil

- 1 tbsp. of maple syrup

- 1/8 tsp of ground cloves

- 3 moderate-sized apples, roughly chopped

- 3 moderate-sized tomatoes, roughly chopped

Directions:

1. Put oil into a huge deep cooking pan and heat it up on moderate heat.

2. Put in shallot and cook until light brown for approximately 2 minutes.

3. Stir in the tomato paste, garlic, salt, pepper, and cloves for approximately half a minute. Then put in in the apples, tomatoes, vinegar, and maple syrup. 4. Bring to its boiling point then decrease the heat to allow it to simmer for approximately 30 minutes. Allow to cool for twenty additional minutes before placing the mixture into your blender. Combine the mixture until the desired smoothness is achieved.

5. Keep in a mason jar or an airtight container; place in your fridge for maximum 5 days.

6. Serve it on a burger or with fries.

Nutritional Info: , Calories: 142 kcal , Protein: 3 g , Fat: 3.46 g , Carbohydrates: 26.93 g

60.   BALSAMIC VINAIGRETTE

Time To Prepare: ten minutes

Time to Cook: 0 minutes **Yield:** Servings 2-4

Ingredients:

- ¼ tsp of freshly ground black pepper

- ½ cup of extra-virgin olive oil

- ½ cup of rice vinegar

- 1 clove of freshly minced garlic

- 1 tbsp. of honey or maple syrup

- 1 tsp of sea or kosher salt

- 2 tsp of Dijon mustard

Directions:

1. Put all ingredients in a mason jar and cover firmly. Shake thoroughly until all ingredients are blended.

2. Keep in your fridge for minimum 30 minutes before you serve to keep its freshness.

3. Serve with a salad or as your meat marinate.

Nutritional Info: , Calories: 147 kcal , Protein: 1.85 g , Fat: 13.21 g , Carbohydrates: 4.02 g

61.   BEAN POTATO SPREAD

Time To Prepare: twenty-five minutes

Time to Cook: 0 minutes **Yield:** Servings 7-8 **Ingredients:**

- ¼ cup sesame paste

- ½ teaspoon cumin, ground

- 1 cup garbanzo beans, drained and washed

- 1 tablespoon olive oil

- 2 tablespoons lime juice

- 2 tablespoons water

- 4 cups cooked sweet potatoes, peeled and chopped

- 5 garlic cloves, minced

- A pinch of salt

Directions:

1. Throw all the ingredients into a blender and blend to make a smooth mix.

2. Move to a container.

3. Serve with carrot, celery, or veggie sticks.

Nutritional Info: Calories 156 , Fat: 3g , Carbohydrates: 10g , Fiber: 6g , Protein: 8g

62.   CASHEW GINGER DIP

Time To Prepare: five minutes

Time to Cook: 0 minutes **Yield:** Servings 1

Ingredients:

• ¼ cup filtered water

• ¼ teaspoon salt

• ½ teaspoon ground ginger

• 1 cup cashews, soaked in water for about twenty minutes and drained

• 1 tablespoon extra-virgin olive oil

• 1 teaspoon lemon juice

• 2 garlic cloves

• 2 teaspoons coconut aminos

• Pinch cayenne pepper

Directions:

1. In a blender or food processor, put together the cashews, garlic, water, olive oil, aminos, lemon juice, ginger, salt, and cayenne pepper. Put in the mix in a container.

2. Cover and place in your fridge until chilled. You can use store it for 4-5 days in your fridge.

Nutritional Info: Calories 124 , Fat: 9g , Carbohydrates: 5g , Fiber: 1g , Protein: 3g

63.   CREAMY AVOCADO DRESSING

Time To Prepare: ten minutes

Time to Cook: 0 minutes **Yield:** Servings 2-4

Ingredients:

- ½ cup of extra-virgin olive oil

- 1 clove of garlic, chopped

- 1 tsp of honey or maple syrup

- 2 small or 1 large-sized avocado, pitted and chopped

- 2 tsp of lemon or lime juice

- 3 tbsp. of chopped parsley

- 3 tbsp. of red wine vinegar

- Onion powder

- Some Kosher salt and ground black pepper

Directions:

1.   Combine all ingredients into a blender, apart from the oil. As the ingredients are mixed, progressively put in the oil into the mixture. Blend until the desired smoothness is achieved or becomes liquidy.

2.   Use as a vegetable or fruit salad dressing. Put in your fridge for maximum 5 days.

Nutritional Info: , Calories: 300 kcal , Protein: 4.09 g , Fat: 27.9 g , Carbohydrates: 11.41 g

64. CREAMY HOMEMADE GREEK DRESSING

Time To Prepare: ten minutes

Time to Cook: 0 minutes **Yield:** Servings 2-4

Ingredients:

- ¼ cup non-dairy milk (e.g., almond, rice milk)

- ½ cup of high-quality mayonnaise, without preservatives

- ½ tsp dried basil

- ½ tsp dried oregano

- ½ tsp parsley

- ½ tsp thyme

- 1/3 cup of extra-virgin olive oil

- 1/4 cup of white wine vinegar

- 2 cloves of garlic, minced

- 2 tbsp. of lemon or lime juice 2 tsp of honey

- A few tablespoons of water • Some Kosher salt and pepper

Directions:

1. Put all together ingredients in a mason jar and shake, cover firmly, and shake thoroughly. Place in your fridge for a few hours before you serve or serve instantly on your favorite vegetable or fruit salad.

2. Shake well before use. Put in your fridge for maximum 5 days.

3. You may put in a few tablespoons of water to tune the consistency as per your preference.

Nutritional Info: , Calories: 474 kcal , Protein: 2.08 g , Fat: 50.1 g , Carbohydrates: 5.31 g

65.   CREAMY RASPBERRY VINAIGRETTE

Time To Prepare: ten minutes

Time to Cook: 0 minutes **Yield:** Servings 2-4

Ingredients:

- ½ cup of raspberries

- 1 tbsp. of Dijon mustard

- 1 tbsp. of Greek yogurt

- 1/3 cup of extra-virgin olive oil

- 2 tbsp. of honey or maple syrup

- 2 tbsp. of raspberry vinegar

Directions:

1.   Put all together the ingredients apart from the oil into a blender, in accordance with the ordered list.

Cover and blend for ten seconds, by slowly increasing the speed.

2.   After 10 seconds, reduce the speed and progressively put in the oil into the mixture. Keep the speed at a stable pace until all of the oil has been poured in. Blend until blended.

3.   Store in a mason jar then place in your fridge for maximum 5 days. Serve with a vegetable or fruit salad.

Nutritional Info: , Calories: 151 kcal , Protein: 2.22 g , Fat: 9.47 g , Carbohydrates: 14.65 g

66.   CREAMY SIAMESE DRESSING

Time To Prepare: ten minutes

Time to Cook: 0 minutes **Yield:** Servings 2-4

Ingredients:

• ¼ cup of non-dairy milk (e.g., almond, rice, soymilk)

• ¼ cup of unsweetened peanut sauce

• 1 cup of mayonnaise

• 1 tbsp. of honey or maple syrup

• 1 tbsps. freshly chopped cilantro

• 2 tbsp. of unsalted peanuts

• 2 tbsp. rice vinegar

Directions:

1. Put all ingredients apart from the cilantro and peanuts into a blender and blend until the desired smoothness is achieved and creamy. Next, put in in the cilantro and peanuts and pulse the blender a few times until completely crushed and well blended. Put in a mason jar and bring it in your fridge.

2. Serve with a garden salad, pasta or as a dipping sauce.

Nutritional Info: , Calories: 525 kcal , Protein: 18.14 g , Fat: 45.55 g , Carbohydrates: 11.01 g

67. CUCUMBER AND DILL SAUCE

Time To Prepare: ten minutes

Time to Cook: 0 minutes **Yield:** Servings 2-4 **Ingredients:**

- ¼ cup of lemon juice

- 1 cucumber, peeled and squeezed to remove surplus liquid

- 1 cup of freshly chopped dill

- 1 tsp of sea salt • 450g of Greek yogurt

Directions:

1. In a moderate-sized container, put together the yogurt, cucumber, and dill then stir until well blended. Put in in the lemon juice and salt to taste.

2. Cover and place in your fridge for approximately 1-2 hours before you serve to keep its freshness. Best serve with Mediterranean food, chips, fish, or even bread.

Nutritional Info: , Calories: 97 kcal , Protein: 13.49 g , Fat: 2.1 g , Carbohydrates: 6.34 g

68. DAIRY-FREE CREAMY TURMERIC DRESSING

Time To Prepare: ten minutes

Time to Cook: 0 minutes **Yield:** Servings 2-4

Ingredients:

- ½ cup of extra-virgin olive oil

- ½ cup of tahini

- 1 tbsp. of turmeric powder

- 2 tbsp. of lemon juice

- 2 tsp of honey

- Some sea salt and pepper

Directions:

1. In a container, whisk all ingredients until well blended.

2. Store in a mason jar and place in your fridge for maximum 5 days.

Nutritional Info: , Calories: 328 kcal , Protein: 7.3 g , Fat: 29.36 g , Carbohydrates: 12.43 g

69. HERBY RAITA

Time To Prepare: ten minutes

Time to Cook: 0 minutes **Yield:** Servings 2-4

Ingredients:

- ¼ cup of freshly chopped mint

- ¼ tsp of freshly ground black pepper

- ½ tsp of sea salt

- 1 cup of Greek yogurt

- 1 large-sized cucumber, shredded

- 1 tsp of lemon juice

Directions:

1.   Combine the cucumber with ¼ tsp of salt in a sieve and leave to drain for fifteen minutes. Shake to release any surplus liquid and move to a kitchen towel. Squeeze out as much liquid as you can using the paper towel.

2.   Put the cucumber into a medium container then mix in the rest of the ingredients until well blended.

3.   Put in your fridge for minimum 2 hours to keep its freshness. Best consume with spicy foods as it could relief the spiciness.

Nutritional Info: , Calories: 69 kcal , Protein: 4.33 g , Fat: 3.66 g , Carbohydrates: 4.93 g

70.   HOMEMADE GINGER DRESSING

Time To Prepare: ten minutes

Time to Cook: 0 minutes **Yield:** Servings 2-4

Ingredients:

- ¼ cup of chopped celery

- ¼ cup of honey or maple syrup

- ¼ cup of water

- ½ cup of chopped carrots

- ½ tsp of white pepper

- 1 cup of chopped onion

- 1 cup of extra-virgin olive oil

- 1 tsp of freshly minced garlic

- 1 tsp of kosher salt

- 2 ½ tbsp. of unsalted, gluten-free soy sauce

- 2 tbsp. of ketchup

- 2/3 cup of rice vinegar • 6 tbsp. of freshly grated ginger

Directions:

1.   Put the onion, ginger, celery, carrots, and garlic into a blender. Blend until the mixture are fine but still lumpy from the small vegetable chunks.

2. Put in in the vinegar, water, ketchup, soy sauce, honey or maple syrup, lemon juice, salt, and pepper. Pulse until the ingredients are well blended. 3. Slowly put in the oil while blending, until everything is thoroughly combined. The mixture must be runny but still grainy.

4. Serve with a winter salad.

Nutritional Info: , Calories: 389 kcal , Protein: 2.71 g , Fat: 32.08 g , Carbohydrates: 22.14 g

71.   HOMEMADE LEMON VINAIGRETTE

Time To Prepare: ten minutes

Time to Cook: 0 minutes **Yield:** Servings 2-4

Ingredients:

• ¼ tsp of sea salt

• ½ tsp of Dijon mustard, without preservatives

• ½ tsp of lemon zest

• 1 tsp of honey or maple syrup

• 2 tbsp. of freshly squeezed lemon juice

• 3 tbsp. of extra-virgin olive oil

• Freshly ground black pepper

Directions:

1. Whisk all together the ingredients apart from olive oil and black pepper in a small container. Then progressively put in 3 tbsp. of olive oil while continuously whisking until well blended. Put in some ground black pepper to taste. Put mason jar and place in your fridge for maximum 3 days. Serve with a garden salads.

Nutritional Info: , Calories: 68 kcal , Protein: 1.69 g , Fat: 6.06 g , Carbohydrates: 1.71 g

72.　　HOMEMADE RANCH

Time To Prepare: ten minutes

Time to Cook: 0 minutes

Yield: Servings 2-4

Ingredients:

- ¼ cup of Greek yogurt

- ¼ tsp Kosher salt

- ½ cup of natural mayonnaise, without preservatives

- ½ tsp of dried dill

- ½ tsp of dried parsley

- ½ tsp of garlic powder

- ½ tsp of onion powder

- ¾ cup of non-dairy milk

- 1/8 tsp Freshly ground black pepper

- 2 tsp of dried chives

Directions:

1. Combine all ingredients apart from the milk into a medium container. Mix together until well blended.

2. Put in in the milk and mix thoroughly.

3. Pour in a mason jar or an airtight container. Serve instantly or place in your fridge for maximum 2 hours to keep the freshness. Put in your refrigerator for maximum 5 days.

4. Serve with a garden or fruit salad.

Nutritional Info: , Calories: 482 kcal , Protein: 3.55 g , Fat: 51.98 g , Carbohydrates: 1.63 g

73.   HONEY BEAN DIP

Time To Prepare: five minutes

Time to Cook: 0 minutes **Yield:** Servings 3-4 **Ingredients:**

- ¼ teaspoon ground cumin

- ¼ teaspoon salt

- 1 (14-ounce) can each of kidney beans and black beans

- 1 tablespoon apple cider vinegar

- 1 teaspoon lime juice

- 2 cherry tomatoes

- 2 garlic cloves

- 2 tablespoons filtered water

- 2 teaspoons raw honey

- Freshly ground black pepper to taste

- Pinch cayenne pepper to taste

Directions:

1. In a blender or food processor, put together the beans, garlic, tomatoes, water, vinegar, honey, lime juice, cumin, salt, cayenne pepper, and black pepper.

2. Blend until it becomes smooth. Put in the mix in a container.

3. Cover and place in your fridge to chill. You can place in your fridge for maximum 5 days.

Nutritional Info: Calories 158 , Fat: 1g , Carbohydrates: 33g , Fiber: 8g , Protein: 9g

74. SOY WITH HONEY AND GINGER GLAZE

Time To Prepare: ten minutes

Time to Cook: 0 minutes **Yield:** Servings 2-4

Ingredients:

- ¼ cup of honey

- 1 tbsp. of rice vinegar

- 1 tsp of freshly grated ginger

- 2 tbsp. gluten-free soy sauce

Directions:

1. Put all together the ingredients into a small container and whisk well.

2. Serve with a vegetables, chickens, or seafood.

3. Keep the glaze in a mason jar, firmly covered, and place in your fridge for maximum four days.

Nutritional Info: , Calories: 90 kcal , Protein: 2.32 g , Fat: 1.54 g , Carbohydrates: 17.99 g

75. STRAWBERRY POPPY SEED DRESSING

Time To Prepare: ten minutes

Time to Cook: 0 minutes **Yield:** Servings 2-4

Ingredients:

• ¼ cup of raspberry vinegar

• ¼ tsp of ground ginger

• ¼ tsp of sea salt ½ tsp of onion powder

• ½ tsp of poppy seeds

• 1/3 cup of extra-virgin olive oil

• 1/3 cup of honey 2 tbsp. of freshly squeezed orange juice

Directions:

1. Put all ingredients, apart from the poppy seeds and oil into a blender. Blend until the desired smoothness is achieved and creamy. Next, progressively put the oil into the mixture until blended. Put in in the poppy seeds and stir thoroughly.

2. Put in a mason jar then place in your fridge before you serve. Keep for maximum 3 days.

3. Serve with your garden salads.

Nutritional Info: , Calories: 167 kcal , Protein: 1.84 g , Fat: 9.35 g , Carbohydrates: 18.89 g

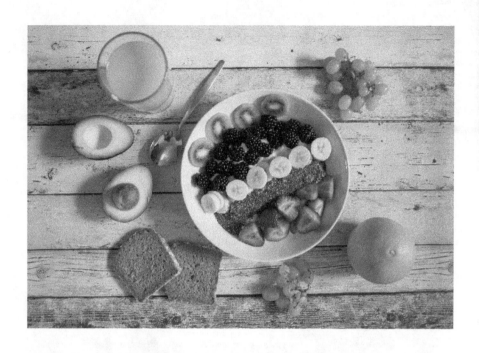

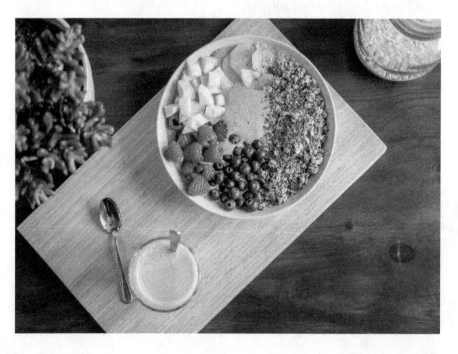

76.   TAHINI DIP

Time To Prepare: ten minutes

Time to Cook: 0 minutes **Yield:** Servings 2-4

Ingredients:

- ¼ cup of tahini

- ½ tsp of maple syrup

- 1 small grated or thoroughly minced clove of garlic (this is optional)

- 1 tbsp. of apple cider vinegar

- 1 tbsp. of freshly squeezed lemon juice

- 1 tbsp. of tamari

- 1 tsp of finely grated ginger, or ½ tsp of ground ginger

- 1 tsp of turmeric

- 1/3 cup of water

Directions:

1. Blend or whisk all ingredients together. Place the dressing in an airtight container then place in your fridge for approximately 5 days.

2. Enjoy!

Nutritional Info: , Calories: 120 kcal , Protein: 4.77 g , Fat: 9.63 g , Carbohydrates: 5.12 g

77.   TOMATO AND MUSHROOM SAUCE

Time To Prepare: ten minutes

Time to Cook: 0 minutes

Yield: Servings 2-4

Ingredients:

- ½ cup of water

- 1 moderate-sized leek, chopped

- 2 moderate-sized carrots, chopped

- 2 stalks of celery, chopped

- 2 tsp of dried oregano

- 4 cloves of garlic, crushed

- 450g of button mushrooms, diced

- 5 tbsp. of coconut milk

- 680g of unsalted tomato puree

- Black pepper, seasoning • Some sea salt, seasoning

Directions:

1.   In a big frying pan, place a few tablespoons of water and heat on moderate heat. Once it sizzles, put in in the mushrooms and Sautee for approximately five minutes, stir once in a while.

2.   Next, put in in the leek, carrots, and celery. Stir thoroughly and cook for approximately five minutes or until the vegetables are soft. Put in more water if required.

3.   Mix in the tomato puree with ½ cup of water and dried oregano. Bring to its boiling point and then decrease the heat to allow it to simmer for approximately fifteen minutes.

4.   Remove from heat and mix in the garlic, coconut milk, and salt and pepper to taste.

5.   Put in an airtight container, then store for maximum four days in your fridge or freeze for maximum 1 month. Serve with a pasta.

Nutritional Info: , Calories: 467 kcal , Protein: 16.91 g , Fat: 3.81 g , Carbohydrates: 109.68 g

78.   ALMOND AND HONEY HOMEMADE BAR

Time To Prepare: fifteen minutes + thirty minutes refrigerator time

Time to Cook: fifteen minutes **Yield:** Servings 8

Ingredients:

- ¼ cup almond butter

- ¼ cup honey

- ¼ cup sugar (or another sweetener to your taste in adjusted amount)

- ¼ cup sunflower seeds

- ½ teaspoon vanilla extract

- 1 cup oats

- 1 cup whole-grain puffed cereal (unsweetened)

- 1 tbsp. flaxseeds

- 1 tbsp. sesame seeds

- 1/3 cup apricots (dried and chopped)

- 1/3 cup currants

- 1/3 cup raisins (chopped)

- 1/8 tsp salt

- A ¼ cup of almonds

Directions:

1. Preheat your oven to 350 degrees Fahrenheit.

2. Place a baking paper to an 8-inch pan or coat it with cooking spray/oil.

3. Combine the almonds, oats, and seeds and spread the mixture on a rimmed baking sheet.

4. Bake the mixture until you notice that the oats are mildly toasted (for approximately ten minutes).

5. Move the mixture to a container.

6. Put in cereal, raisins, currants, and apricots to the container.

7. Toss thoroughly to blend.

8. Mix honey, almond butter, vanilla, salt, and sugar in a deep cooking pan. 9. Heat on moderate heat. Stir regularly for 2-5 minutes until you see light bubbles.

10. Once you notice the bubbles, pour the mixture over the dry mixture with apricots and oats you prepared previously.

11. Mix thoroughly using a spatula. There mustn't be any dry spots.

12. Move the new mixture to the previously prepared pan.

13. Push it to the pan to make a firm and flat layer.

14. Place in your refrigerator for half an hour

15. Chop the layer into eight equal bars or squares, to your taste.

16. Consume instantly or place in your refrigerator up to seven days.

Nutritional Info: , Calories: 213 kcal , Protein: 6.92 g , Fat: 9.59 g , Carbohydrates: 32.33 g

79. ALMONDS AND BLUEBERRIES YOGURT SNACK

Time To Prepare: ten minutes

Time to Cook: 0 minutes **Yield:** Servings 2

Ingredients:

• 1 ½ cups nonfat Greek yogurt

• 1 cup blueberries • 20 almonds, chopped

Directions:

1. Take 2 bowls and put in ¾ cup yogurt into each container.

2. Split the blueberries among the bowls and stir.

3. Drizzle half the almonds in each container before you serve.

Nutritional Info: , Calories: 223 kcal , Protein: 6.57 g , Fat: 9.45 g , Carbohydrates: 30.82 g

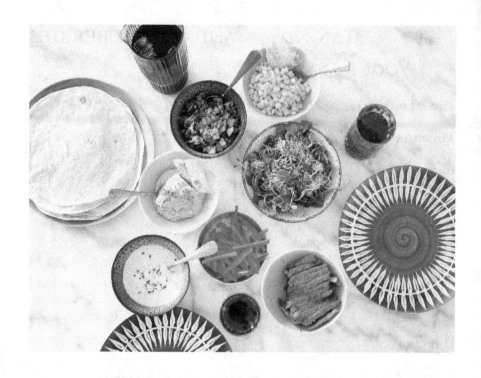

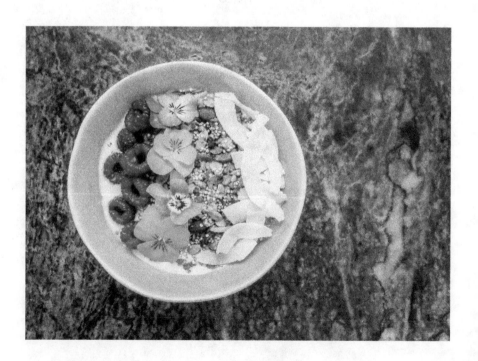

80.   ANTI-INFLAMMATORY KEY LIME PIE

Time To Prepare: twenty minutes + thirty-five minutes refrigerator time **Time to Cook:** 0 **Yield:** Servings 8

Ingredients:

- ½ cup honey

- ½ cup Medjool dates, chopped and pitted

- 1 cup unsweetened shredded coconut

- 1 cup walnuts

- 1 teaspoon lime zest

- 1/4 teaspoon sea salt

- 3 firm avocados

- 3 tablespoons lime juice

- Lime slices

- Pinch of sea salt

Directions:

1.   Use a food processor to put all together the walnuts, coconut, and the salt, then pulse until crudely ground.

2.   Place the dates and pulse until the mixture resembles bread crumbs, trying to stick together.

3. Push the mixture into the edges and bottom of a non-stick greased 9-inch pie pan. Use your fingers or the back of a spoon to press the crust into a uniform layer. Bring the crust into the freezer for minimum fifteen minutes while preparing the filling.

4. Use the food processor again and mix the avocado, honey, lime juice, lime zest, and salt. Process until the desired smoothness is achieved.

5. Pour the filling into the now-chilled piecrust and place it in your fridge for about twenty minutes.

6. Decorate using fresh lime slices and serve cold. Store any left overs in your fridge.

Nutritional Info: , Calories: 273 kcal , Protein: 4.19 g , Fat: 18.4 g , Carbohydrates: 28.49 g

CPSIA information can be obtained
at www.ICGtesting.com
Printed in the USA
BVHW040713220321
603170BV00004B/753